My Body

Martin Skelton and David Playfoot

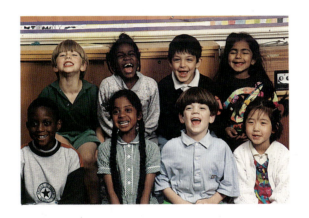

Contents

Busy body

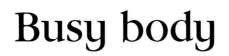

Sam's day

Bodies are always busy.
Sam's body did all these
things yesterday.
It woke up.
It ate breakfast.
It drank some milk.
It looked and listened. It spoke.

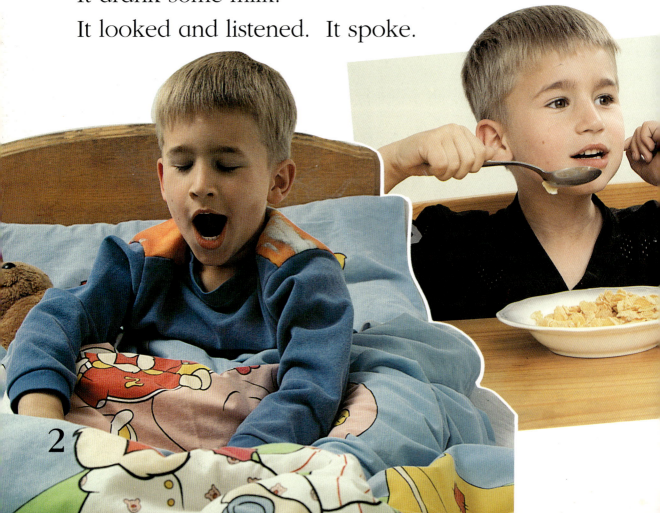

2

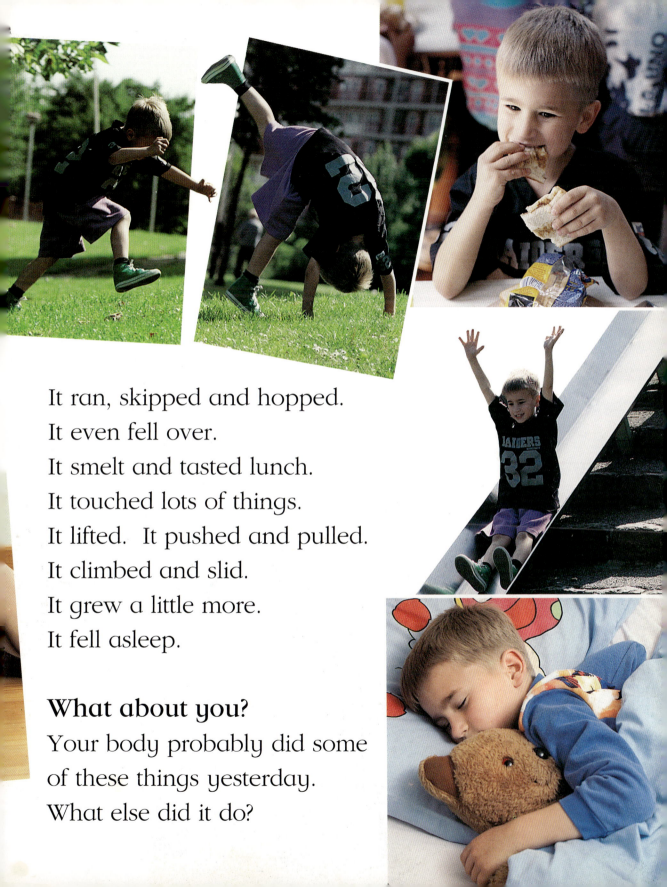

It ran, skipped and hopped.
It even fell over.
It smelt and tasted lunch.
It touched lots of things.
It lifted. It pushed and pulled.
It climbed and slid.
It grew a little more.
It fell asleep.

What about you?

Your body probably did some
of these things yesterday.
What else did it do?

On the outside

Yasmin's body

This is what
Yasmin's body
looks like from
the outside.
Look at all the
different parts of
her body. Can
you find her skin,
hair, eyes, ears,
nose and
mouth?

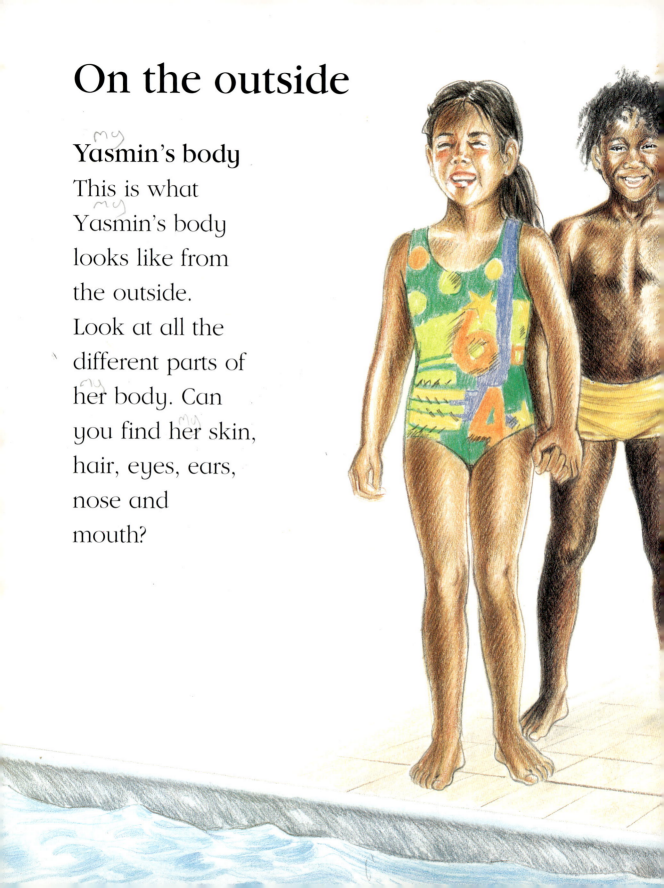

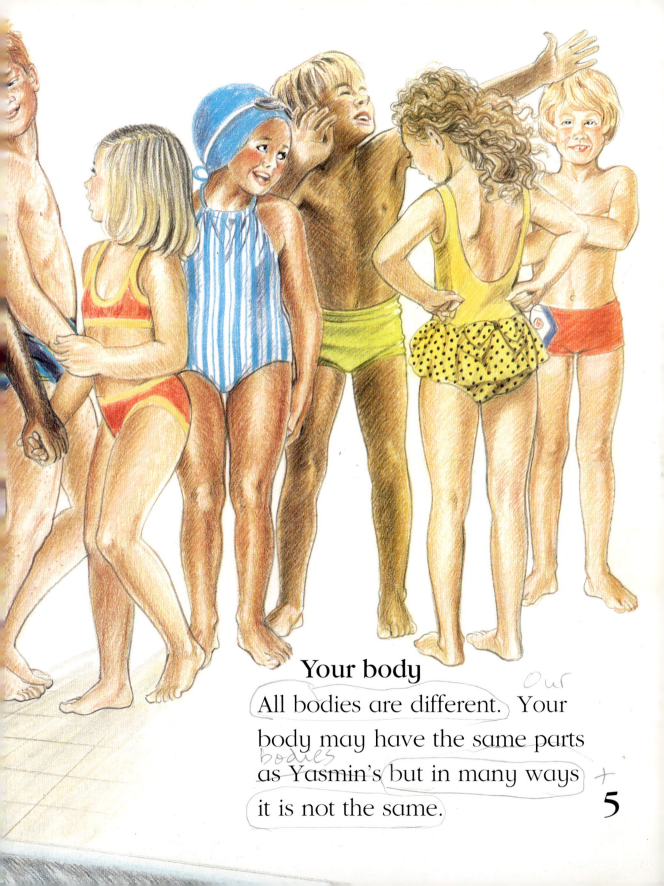

Your body

All bodies are different. Your body may have the same parts as Yasmin's but in many ways it is not the same.

5

On the inside

What's inside?
Your body has many parts on the inside that you cannot see. Here's what Yasmin's body would look like if you could see inside it. You have the same parts inside your body. You can feel some of them from the outside.

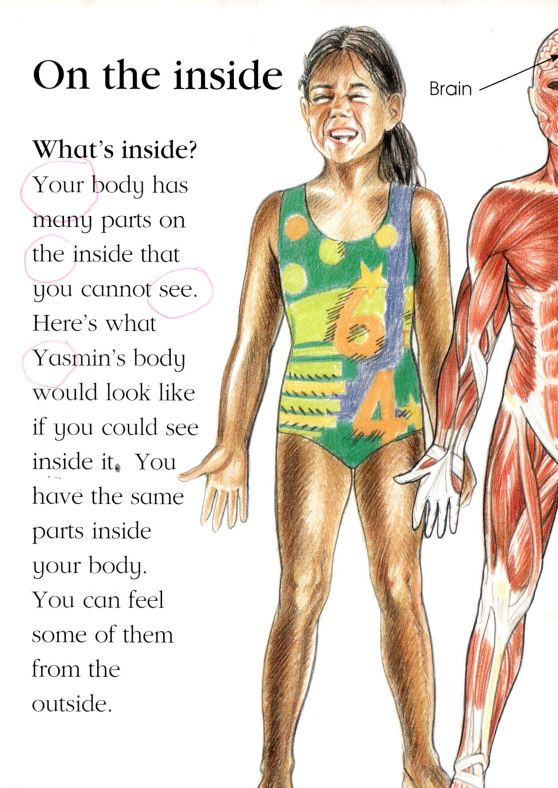

Brain

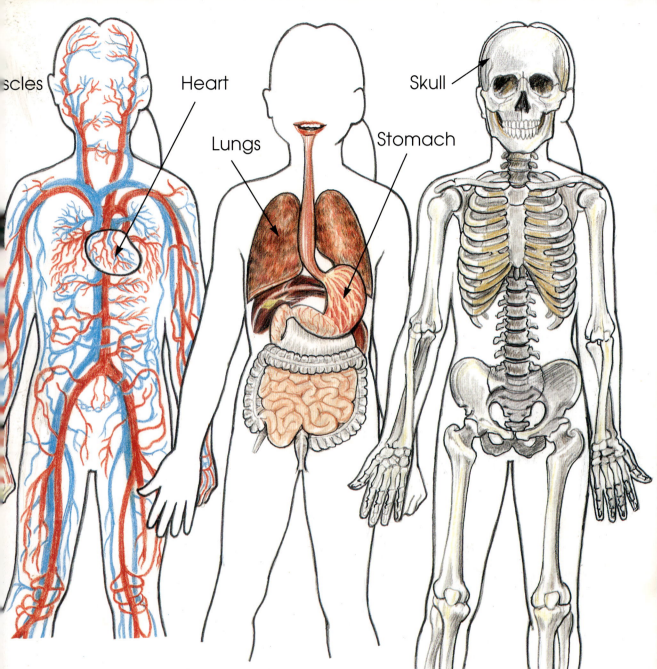

scles

Heart

Lungs

Stomach

Skull

Hard at work

Your body never stops working for a second.
Some parts of your body have just one job to do.
Others do a number of different jobs. And many
parts work together.

7

Skin

Look at your skin

Your skin is soft and thin, but it's very tough. You can pull it, twist it, knock it, squeeze it. Some of your skin is smooth, but on your fingertips it has ridges to help you hold and feel things better.

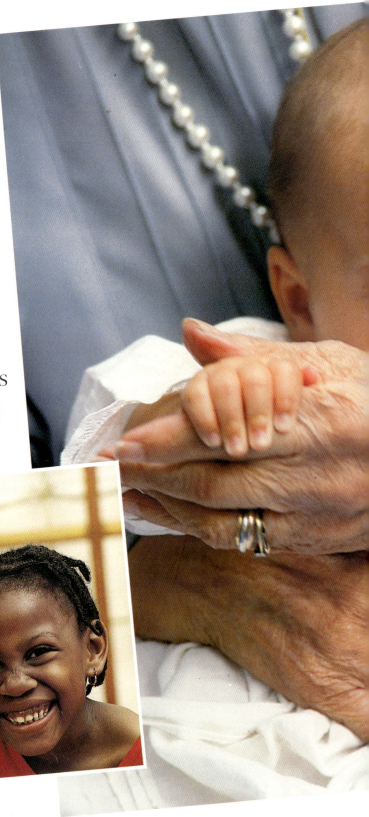

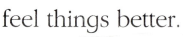

8

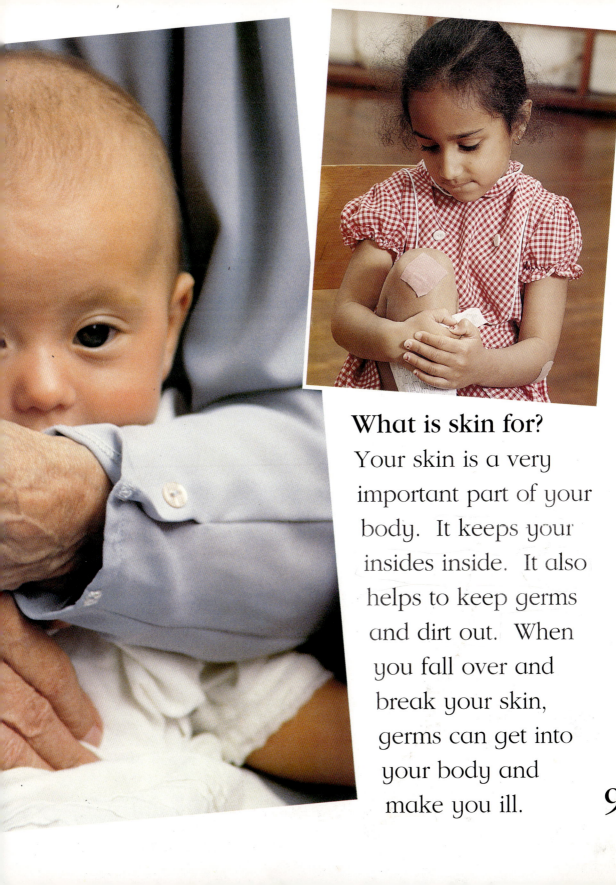

What is skin for?

Your skin is a very
important part of your
body. It keeps your
insides inside. It also
helps to keep germs
and dirt out. When
you fall over and
break your skin,
germs can get into
your body and
make you ill.

9

Hair

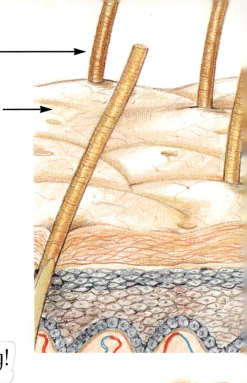

Hair

Skin

Where does hair grow?

Hair grows on your head, of course. It also grows on your skin. Can you see the tiny hairs on your arms and legs? When you're older, hair can grow almost everywhere on your body!

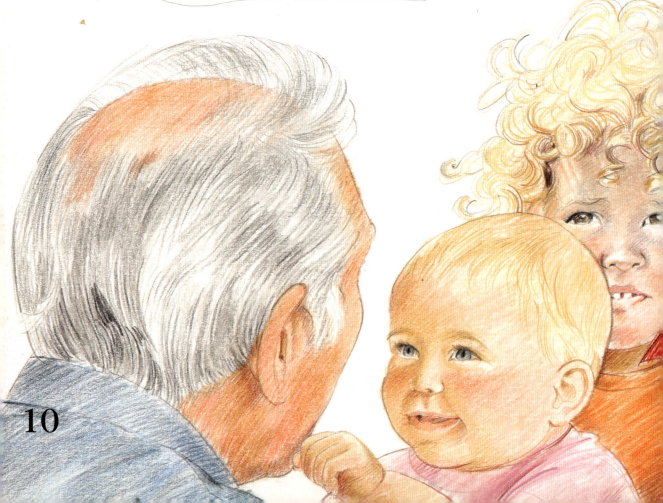

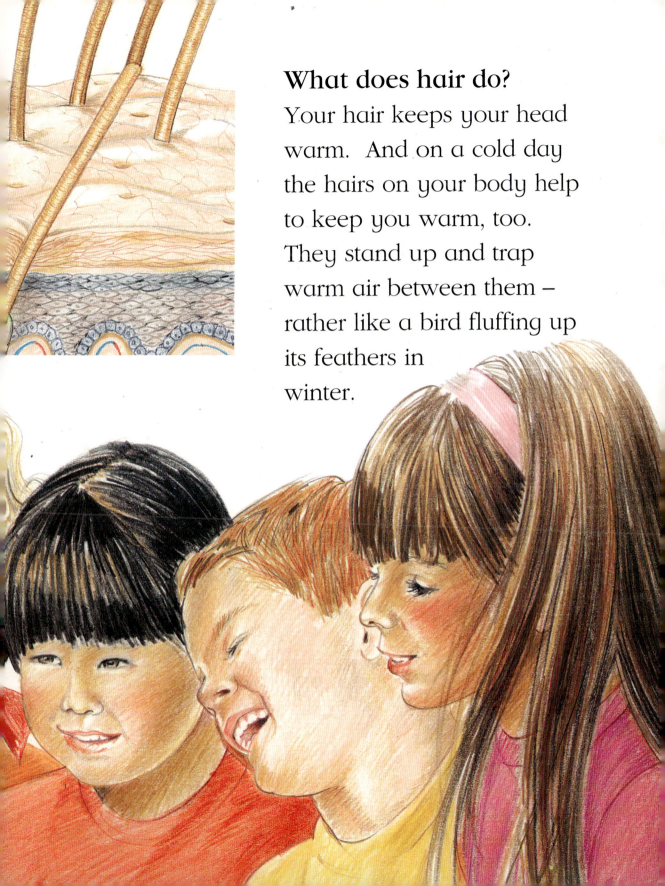

What does hair do?

Your hair keeps your head warm. And on a cold day the hairs on your body help to keep you warm, too. They stand up and trap warm air between them – rather like a bird fluffing up its feathers in winter.

Bones

You have lots of bones in your body. They are all different shapes and sizes. Together they make your skeleton.

What does your skeleton do?

Your skeleton is strong like the frame of a tent. Without it, you'd be floppy like a rag doll. The hard bones also protect the soft, precious parts inside your body like your heart and brain.

12

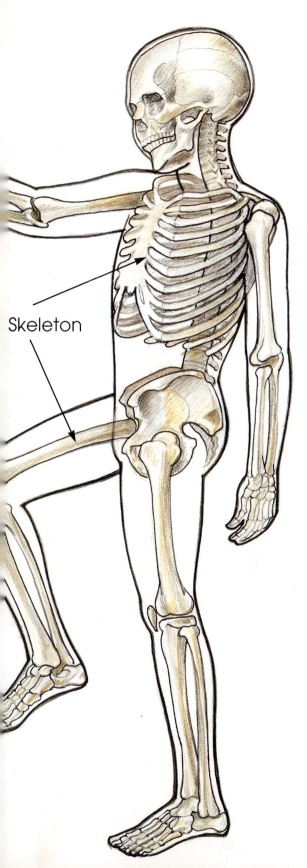

Skeleton

Bones alive!

The bones you see in museums are dry and dead, but inside your body they grow and are alive. Did you know that if you break a bone it can mend itself if it is put back together properly?

Lung

Heart

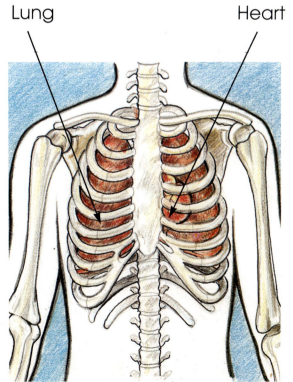

13

Joints

Look at a finger

If you look closely, you will see that your finger is made from three bones. The bones meet in two places, called joints.

What do joints do?

If your fingers were made with one long bone instead of three small ones, they wouldn't be able to bend. It's the joints in your body that help you to bend, turn and jump.

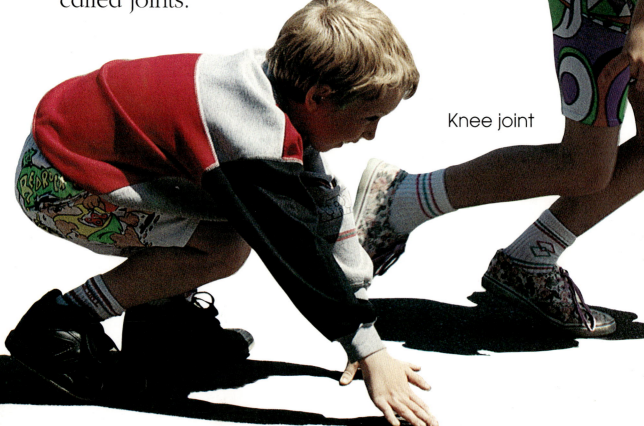

Knee joint

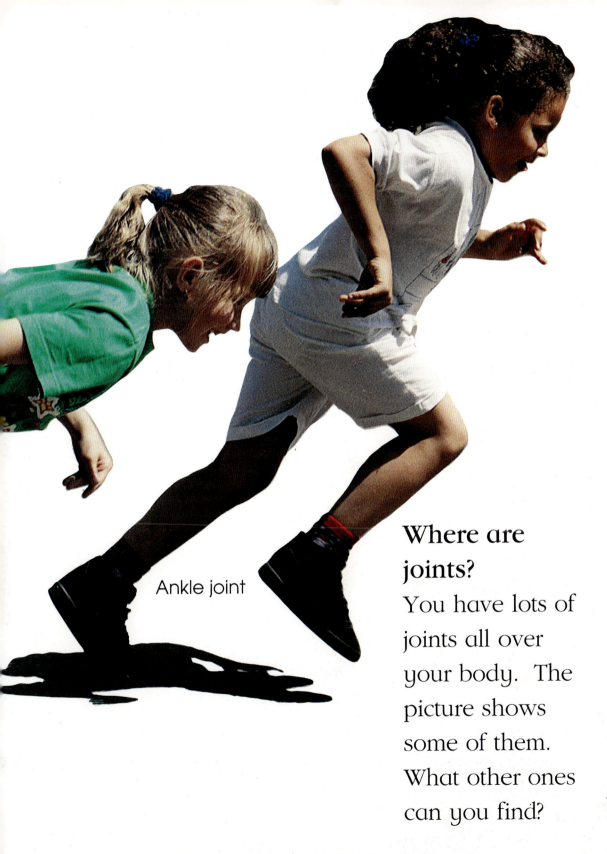

Ankle joint

Where are joints?

You have lots of joints all over your body. The picture shows some of them. What other ones can you find?

15

Muscles

Your bones and joints cannot move on their own. They need muscles.

What do muscles do?

It's your muscles that make your body move and change shape. They pull on your bones and skin so that you can run, smile, stretch – and do all the other things you need to do.

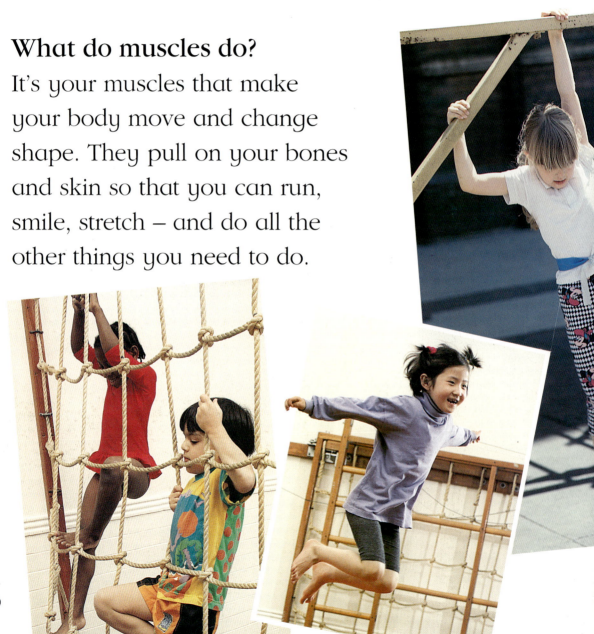

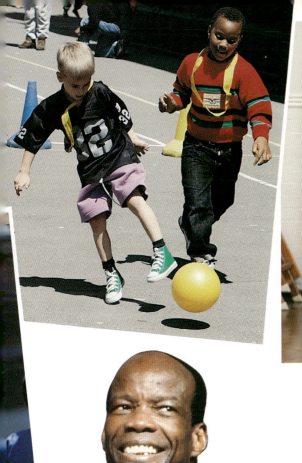

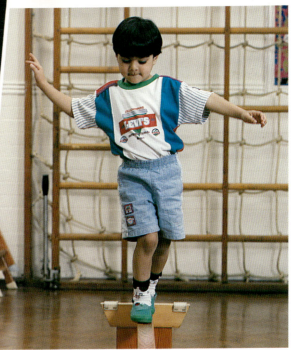

Where are muscles?

Try bending your elbow. Can you feel a bulge in your arm? That's a muscle. You have muscles everywhere in your body – even in your eyes and mouth. And the more you use muscles, the stronger they get.

17

Blood

The blood in your body would fill about seven drink cans. It travels round and round like a train that never stops, along tubes called blood vessels.

How does blood move?

Blood can't move by itself. It's pumped along by a big muscle. That muscle is your heart, and when it pumps, it pushes the blood around your body through the arteries. Blood returns to your heart through the veins.

What does blood do?

Blood carries food and oxygen to every part of your body. And it takes away the waste that your body can't use.

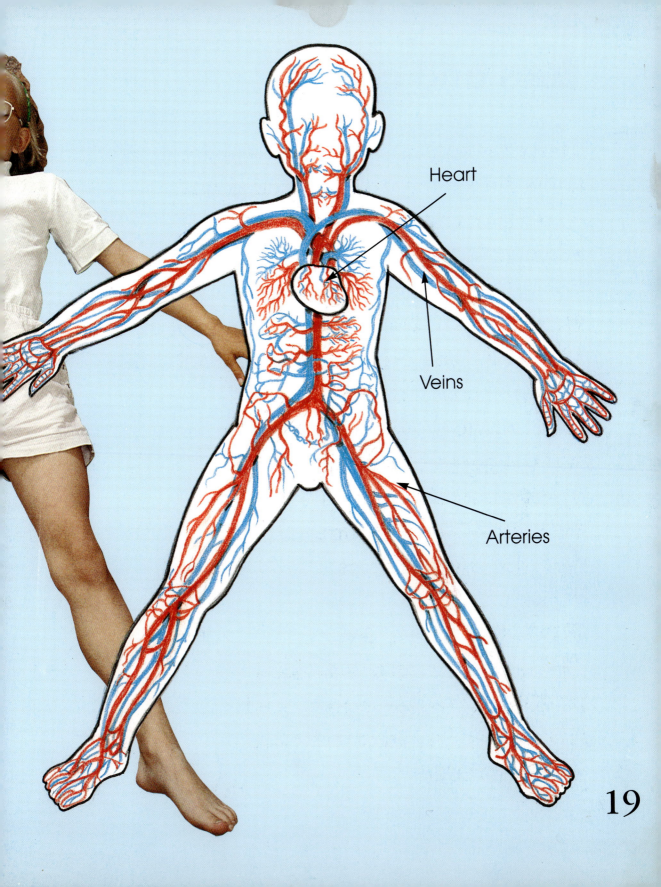

Heart

Veins

Arteries

19

Eyes and ears

Your eyes and ears help you to understand what's happening in the world around you.

Seeing

Your eyes are at the front of your head, right at the top of your body. They can see all around you. Have you ever been blindfolded? Then you will know how important your eyes are. Take care to protect them from the sun.

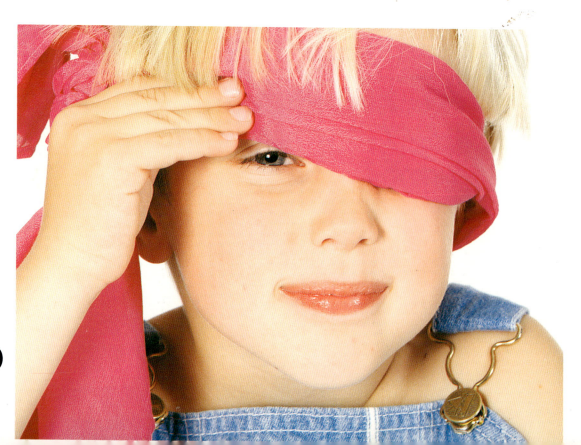

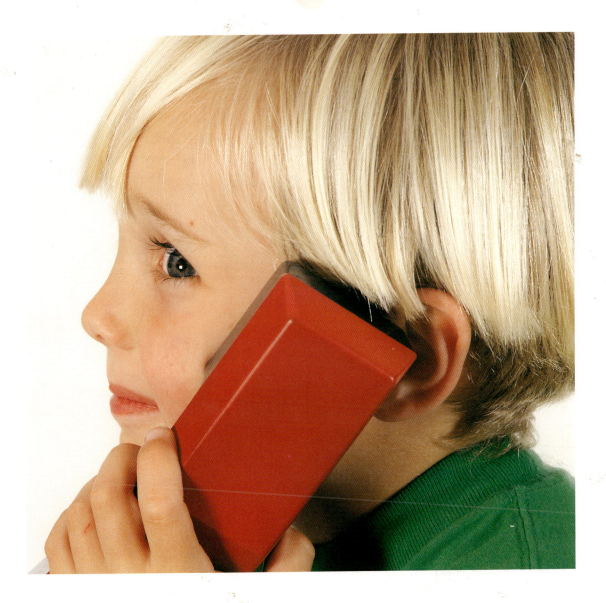

Hearing

The shape of your ear helps you to
pick up as many sounds as possible.
Put your hands over your ears to
block out the sounds around you.
What can you hear now?

21

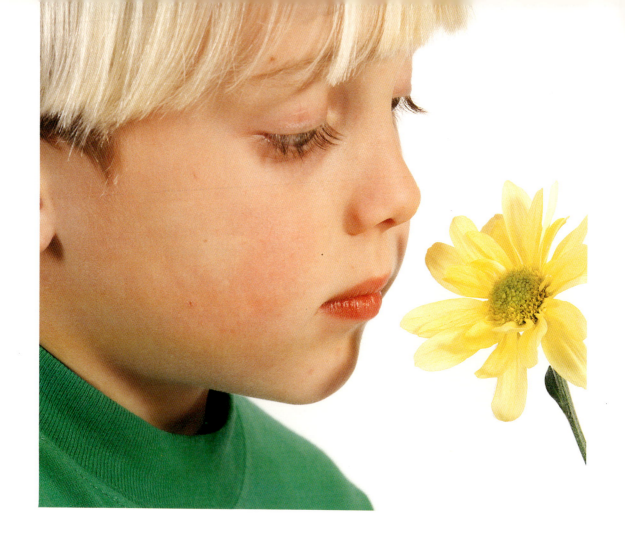

Nose and mouth

Breathing and smelling

Your nose does three important jobs. It takes in
fresh air, which your body needs to live. It has
hairs inside to stop dirt getting into your body.
And, of course, it helps you to smell everything
22 from cabbage to candyfloss!

Tasting

Inside your mouth are your teeth and tongue. Your tongue is a muscle. It helps you to move bits of food around your mouth. It also helps you to taste the foods you eat – sweet, sour, salty or bitter.

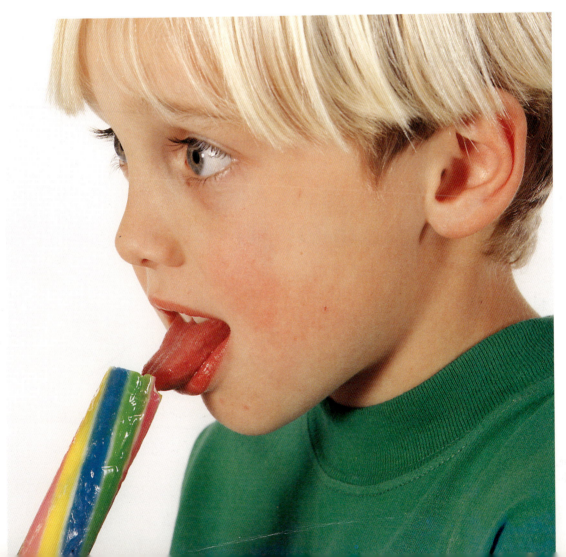

Teeth

Your teeth are hard.
They're for chewing food.

When do teeth grow?
When you were a baby,
you drank lots of milk.
You didn't need teeth.
But soon your teeth
began to grow to let
you eat different
foods.

Look at your teeth
Your front teeth are
sharp like scissors.
They cut your food to
bits. Your back teeth
are flat. They mash
your food, and make
it easy to swallow.

24

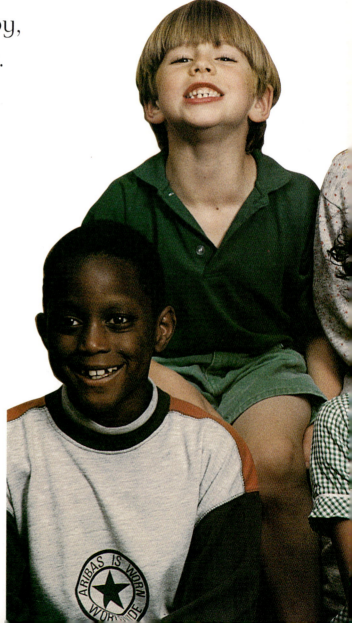

Look after your teeth
Don't eat too many sweets.
Brush your teeth twice a day.
Visit your dentist often.

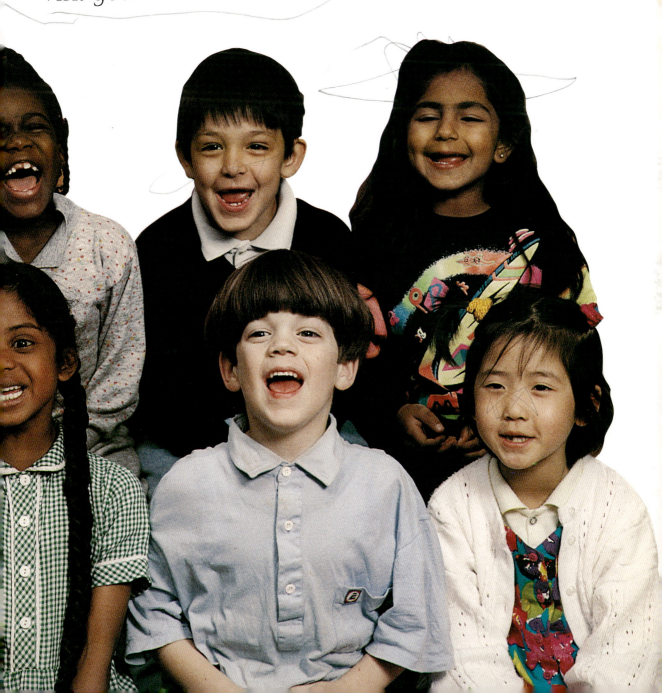

Food

Your body needs a number of different foods. Some foods, like meat, fish and beans help you to grow. Other foods, such as bread and potatoes, give you energy. And others, like fresh fruit and vegetables, keep you healthy, too.

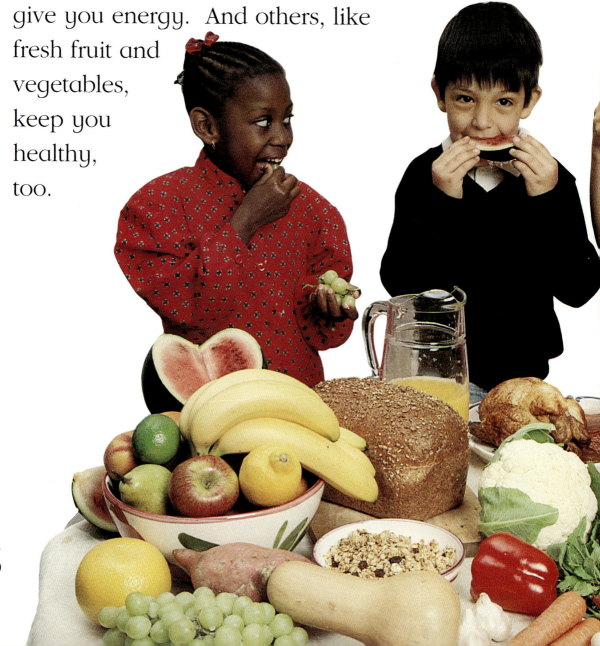

What happens to the food?

The food you eat travels right through your body. Your body takes the goodness out of the food as it moves along – from your mouth, to your stomach, to your intestine. Any food your body can't use comes out when you go to the toilet.

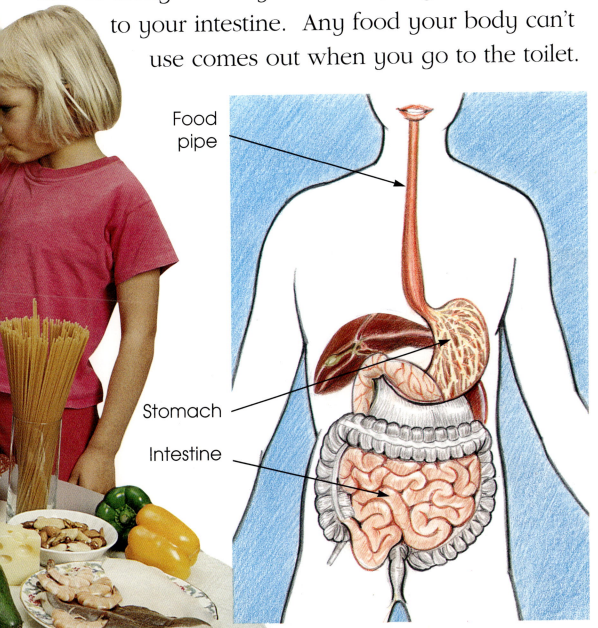

Food pipe

Stomach

Intestine

27

Brain

Where is it?

Your brain lies inside the top of your head.
Because it is soft – and very important – it is
well protected by your hard skull.

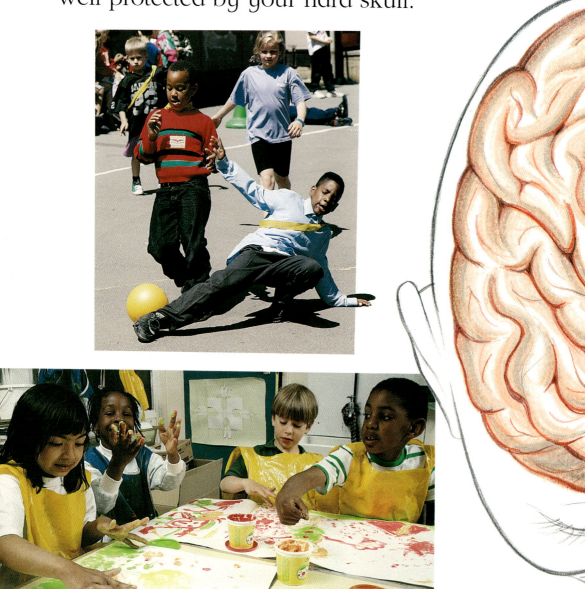

What does it do?

Your brain controls every part of your body. It sorts out the messages from your eyes, ears, nose, mouth and skin. It sends instructions to your heart, lungs, joints and muscles.

Without your brain you wouldn't be able to see, speak, hear or feel. You couldn't think or move.

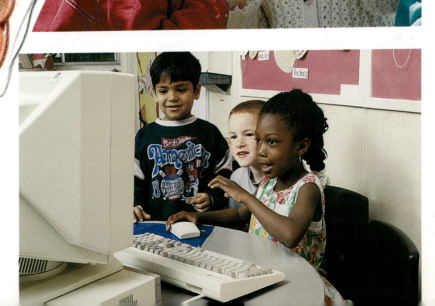

29

A very busy day

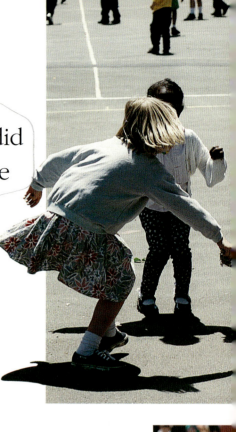

When someone asks you "What did you do today?" tell them you have been very, very busy.

After all…
Your hair grew.
Your teeth cut and chewed food.
Your nose smelled smells.
You took in air.
You took goodness from the food you ate.
Your skin stopped germs getting inside you.
Your skeleton moved hundreds of times.
Your muscles moved your bones.
Your heart pumped blood around your body.
Your brain looked after everything you did.

Yes, you and your body have been
very busy today!

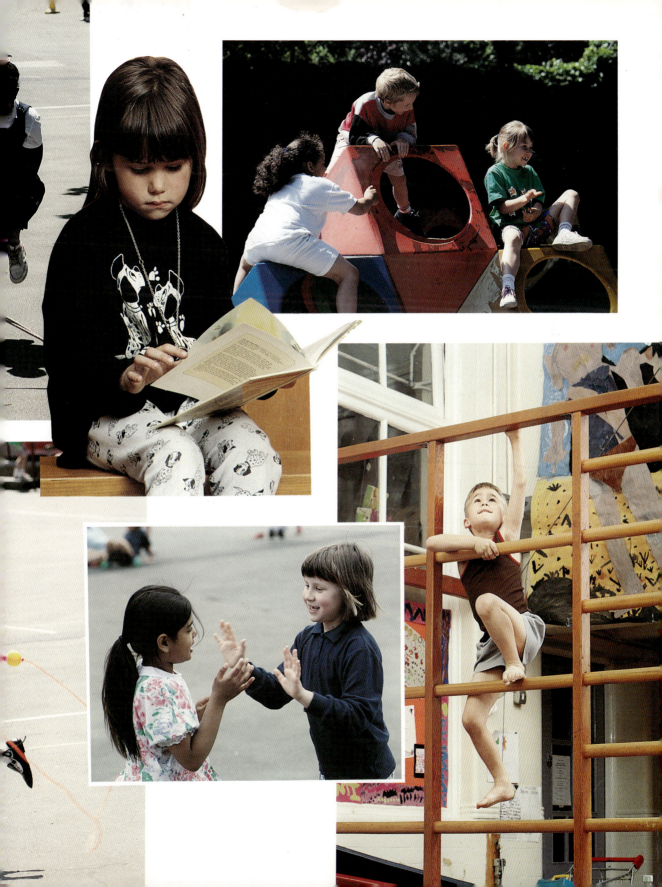

Index

HarperCollins Children's Books

A Division of HarperCollins Publishers Ltd, 77–85 Fulham Palace Road, Hammersmith, London W6 8JB

First published 1994 in the United Kingdom

Copyright © HarperCollins*Publishers* 1994

Prepared by *specialist publishing services* 090 857 307

ISBN 0 00 196540 9

A CIP record is available from the British Library

Printed and bound in Hong Kong

Illustrated by Joan Corlass

Photographs by John Walmsley except pp20/21, pp22/23 by Fiona Pragoff, pp8/9 c Bubbles/Michelle Garret, p17 bc Allsport

Series editor: Nick Hutchins; Editing: Claire Llewellyn; Design: Eric Drewery/Susi Martin;

Picture research: Lorraine Sennett